HBC Matters

How Everything Matters and How to Handle Every Matter in Surviving Hereditary Breast Cancer – My Cancer Survival Story

By

Celia Eloise

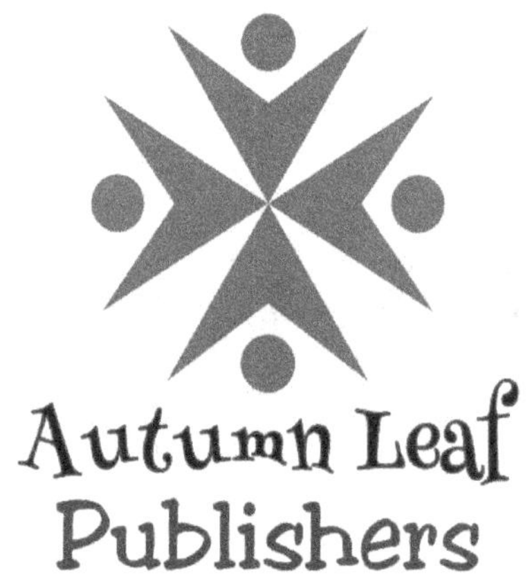

Design & Illustration by Jordy Roberts

First Edition

Disclaimer

This book chronicles the individual experiences of one cancer survivor. The narrative contained herein is not intended to provide diagnosis, treatment advice, or to replace the advice of professionals.

Always consult a doctor or treatment professional for your individual needs. No responsibility is accepted by the author or the publisher for any damages or loss resulting from misinterpretation of the information contained in this book.

Any information in this book is provided as an anecdote or purely for reference purposes. It is not intended to diagnose, treat, or to take the place of advice from a medical professional. Always consult your doctor before undertaking any lifestyle change such as exercise, diet, or utilizing alternative therapies.

Contact information for resources listed is current as of the time of publication and is subject to change.

Contents

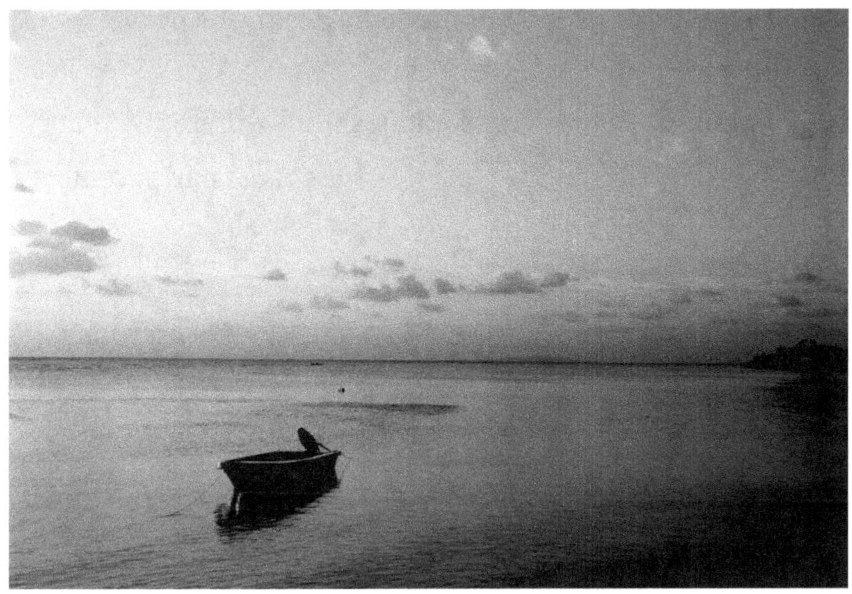

Do you have the cancer gene?

This may seem like a strange question to some, but as it turns out, it is the very inquisition that could save your life.

When I was growing up, characteristics coming from a person's parents were lauded. People would say things like, "Yeah, she's beautiful just like her mother" or "He is as strong as an ox, just like his daddy."

Everything attributed to one's parents was an inherited benefit to their journey through life. This is what I had always known things to be, but never could I have imagined being given something unloving, potentially deadly, or irreversible.

People in the Southern United States think differently than those in other parts of the world. For the most part, events don't just happen out of the blue.

There was always a reason for everything. I grew up where there were always impending storms, hurricanes, and flooding. Living conditions were great until the sky become dark, the wind picked up speed, and whatever you were doing came to a resounding halt.

Stay still.

This will soon come to pass. This was figuratively and literally.

I wondered if I could rely on those early messages from my past to lean on with the storm erupting right before my eyes.

Something just didn't seem right one fateful morning. I didn't know what exactly made me feel off balance. My gut told me something was brewing, and I would soon find out.

My mother had beckoned my presence. A neighbor came over to guide me to my mother's house. I was all over the place with anxiety.

What in the world did she want where she would send someone to find me to rush over to her house? The skin underneath my mother's right armpit was sore and swollen, she said. Still, I thought, nothing that a visit to the doctor's office couldn't fix.

I died that day the doctor told my mother and me that he suspected she had breast cancer and wanted to conduct a biopsy to confirm or rule it out altogether. My mother had noticed a growth of some sort underneath her right armpit, I told the physician who examined her.

I later learned this was her lymph nodes trying to filter out the harmful toxins it detected somewhere in her body.

How could something as small as the tip of an ink pen wreak such havoc?

Cancer was never on our radar - ever. A part of me began to dissipate. I was having an out-of-body experience. That is exactly how I would describe it. I was perceiving my world from another location other than my physical body.

I felt like I was one of those people from the movies who were killed and still roamed the earth. I remember writing a story about those people who were stolen from a hospital, pronounced dead, and scavengers would creep in to take the body for medical experiments.

Despite this nagging doubt that the end may very well be fast-approaching, we were hopeful that the doctors had caught cancer in time to cure it. I sat in on the conversations my mother shared with the physician, his guidance on which way to turn, and what exactly to do next.

He referred several cancer advocates to us, and we explored them all. We equipped ourselves with the education we needed to proceed.

Knowledge is power, and we needed a whole lot of that.

In the coming days, we thought of little else and spoke of little else. When the test results finally came back from the biopsy, the blow was even more troubling than our suspicions.

Once the shock lessened, we decided to take action. We finally shared this information with family members who were equally as confused.

Our church dedicated a Sunday sermon in her honor, and the prayer warriors danced and prayed around her. This took place every single Sunday. Surely, God could see and hear the SOS signals. All we thought we could do at the time was sit on our hands and wait. Waiting has never been a virtue of mine.

I remembered a talk my grandmother gave me about patience when I asked her, "What on earth was taking God's miracle so long to appear?"

She replied, "Just wait on time, baby. Just wait on time."

Just wait on time.

I took a deep breath. My nana was right, I need to calm myself because everything would come in due season.

As time went on and my mother followed the doctor's recommended treatment plan to survive breast cancer, I secretly felt like this was happening to me, too. I never uttered a word about this suffocating feeling.

Somehow the disease had transcended my mother's body onto mine. The disease had changed everything - my attitude towards other people, the activities I participated in, and my everyday routines were dissolving piece by piece, all around me. I escorted my mother to and from her chemotherapy and radiation treatments until they were finally complete.

We were assured that the medical team was doing all it could to destroy the cancer cells in her body. Somewhere, in this mist of pulling at straws and obtaining new information about tackling the illness, came the suggestion of trying alternative therapies to cure the disease.

This meant following an obscure "expert" who was a lay doctor of sorts. This "doctor" may or may not have a Ph.D.

He prescribed a rigid diet of certain foods, supplements, and the complete cessation of all toxins formally put in the body. No salt, so sugar, no cigarettes, and no alcohol.

This regime increased our hope that everything was going to be okay and would be back to normal soon. Slowly, my mother's hair began to shed until she became completely bald. This optic was shocking, to say the least. We purchased a stylish wig, and no one was the wiser in public.

Little by little, my mother began to resume her former activities and routines. It was like she had received a new lease on life. Doctors said the cancer cells had been destroyed after completing the mastectomy and treatment prescribed.

Things went back to as they had been before the news came about the breast cancer. Three years went by, and my mother's remission was in full swing. There were no signs of cancer cells or growth in her system.

We were hit with a piercing blow. The news came that the cancer had returned - and it came back with fierce aggression.

The mutated cells were growing uncontrollably until there was nothing more that could be done. She lost the fight with breast cancer.

Somehow, this didn't make any sense to me. It ran counter to everything I was taught from birth.

Murderers, abusers, rapists, liars, cheaters, gangbangers, and mobsters are free to live, roam the earth, and continue to spread their mayhem, but my sweet, loving mother was sentenced to die because she developed a disease she had no control over.

"Sometimes bad things happen to good people," this old man told me once. This instance must have been what he was speaking of.

Twenty years passed since this fateful moment. The raincloud that formed above my head had finally disappeared. I had almost forgotten that I could even be at risk of contracting the disease until I went for my annual gynecological visit, and the doctor reminded me about my mammogram. I had put it off as long as I could.

At the time, a mammogram was a constant reminder of my previous loss. For me, it wasn't just going to get a mammogram. This required days of mental preparation. I had to prepare myself for whatever these results would reveal.

I had to brace myself for anything.

When I finally did go for the test, the examiners asked me to stay back to talk to the doctor. X-ray imaging found a lump on my breast.

Would I be reliving this nightmare all over again?

My doctor insisted that I seek counseling for any psychological issues that were sure to arise.

Perhaps, if I didn't do anything about it, it would go away. This was a pipe dream, my surgeon explained.

There had been medical advancements made in the twenty years since my first encounter with breast cancer. I finally agreed to go forth with surgery, chemotherapy, radiation, and the treatment plan to cure the cancer.

I didn't feel confident that it would work at all. I was stoic, unfeeling, and could have been an innocent bystander in this whole ordeal.

I played along, followed instructions, and hoped for the best.

I, too, lost my hair, had the surgery to remove the lump, and was sick to my stomach for a while from the aftereffects of the chemotherapy.

I went to work virtually every day and pretended that everything was fine in my world. And for a brief moment, everything was okay.

Doing some activity like working gave me an opportunity to concentrate on something else besides cancer.

I changed my eating habits to natural foods, watched my weight, stayed away from known toxins, and proceeded to take a deep breath again.

Full speed ahead, I thought.

I decided to share my cancer experience with my extended family, hoping this would somehow help me come to grips with the disease if I said it aloud.

The doctors had mentioned that I had Stage II cancer, which had shown previous signs of full recovery with treatment. I participated in their clinical trials and their new medicines. These are often things people typically ran away from, but I thought if my being an experiment would help the next person in this condition, then it was all good to me.

I bought a few wigs and wore make up every day. I had gotten this motivation from my surgeon, who often showed up clad in a white medical robe and pumps.

Her make-up was carefully applied, and she looked like she had just stepped out of a fashion magazine. I thought, "I want to be just like her when I grow up."

As I looked back on this, I remember the first time I laughed again. I was given some popular comedy movies from an up and coming entertainer which became my healing power.

I created an entire business on the foundation of laughter being the best medicine. I hosted events with local comedians and some national ones. I spread the message about breast cancer awareness, and soon I was feeling like my old self again.

Positivity matters.

I practiced affirmations in the bathroom mirror daily. I had said those powerful words so often that I began to believe them in the inside of my soul.

I surrounded myself with positivity in my friends, in my work, and in my personal life. You will eventually have a personal life again.

Look yourself straight in the mirror and tell yourself,"what you see is what you get" and continue to love yourself just the way you are.

Connecting with other people in the same situation with support groups is also a good suggestion. Interacting with other breast cancer survivors removes the feeling of isolation and loneliness that may crop up from time to time.

This is why I have written my experiences in this book. I want to share what I have learned on this journey with others. I want you to know what matters – and that everything matters – when you are surviving hereditary breast cancer.

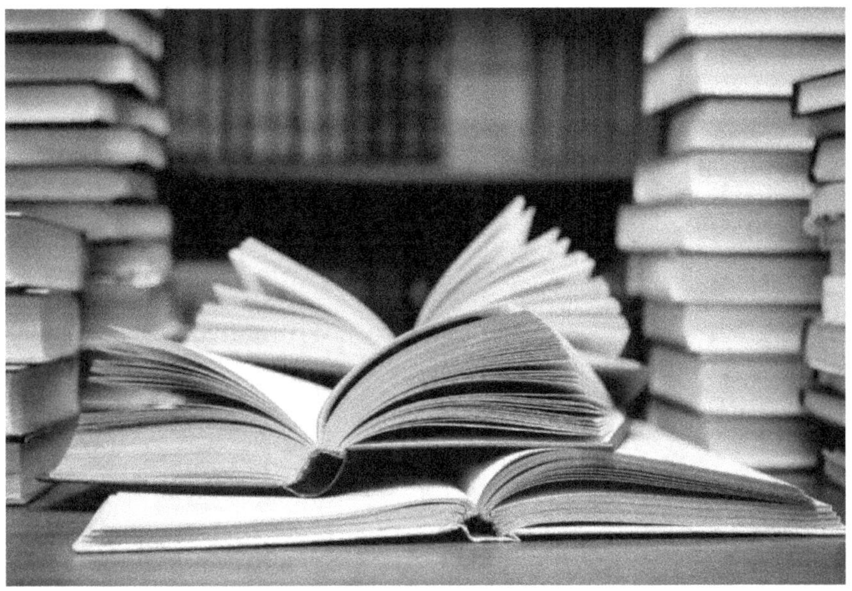

Reflecting on my situation when this matter all started, I had often thought about if my days were numbered. Once the doctor revealed my cancer diagnosis, death was imminent and would come like a thief in the night to suck the very life right out of me.

My mother taught me never to show fear around an adversary or opponent. Look them straight in the eye, don't flinch, and dare them to make the first move. Even if you were shaking in your boots, never let on that you were scared.

I would be meeting my maker soon. I thought of all the things that I had done in my life, even that thing I did in college that I thought the Lord said he had forgiven me for. I couldn't quite put my hand on what would have prompted such traumatizing news. Once I exhausted this list and ended my own personal pity party, I sat and just waited to see what to do next or what would happen next. Everything became a blur at that point.

I remembered reading the phrase,"Darkness defined the light." Despite the way things looked, I would use the cancer as a catalyst to move me forward in life from here on.

I used this devastating disease to launch and carve out a new and improved life for myself and my family. As I began to grow stronger every day, so did my outlook on my future. Instead of cancer defining me, it propelled me forward.

This is not something that I ever remembered my family sitting around the dinner table discussing or openly talking about. A conversation about anything regarding body parts was taboo, shunned, and considered disrespectful from the elders' point of view. Any conversations about the body are done in private, and only after the person you are telling this to is sworn to secrecy - even amongst a trusted audience of other women.

Information was shared over cooking, washing clothes, minding the kids, or doing other household chores usually relegated to women. Cancer was never a subject that emerged out from nowhere or something that had somehow fallen from the sky. All matters about the anatomy were spoken in quiet whispers and never ever when men were around.

Sharing information matters.

I was starting from ground zero in collecting any details about cancer in my personal circle. Delving into my past and the past of other people raised the curtains for me to continue to try to dismantle this shroud of secrecy.

No one was forthcoming. Even I felt like this made me odd, different, and not part of the status quo. Cancer is likened to a shadow that walks around with you. Everywhere you turn, its always there to remind you of its existence. I initially couldn't shake it.

Outside of that state, I decided to educate myself on the matter of cancer. I found out that it all starts with a small collection of cells that mutate or grow uncontrollably and form a tumor. From there, this development sends the body way out whack. The lymph nodes, acting as filters, work to remove and clear this massive collection of harmful cells.

Statistics matter.

Breast cancer is one of the leading causes of death among women. Every year, approximately 252,710 women are diagnosed in this country, and at least 40,500 will ultimately die from the illness.

According to the National Breast Cancer Foundation, Inc.:

- At least one in eight women will experience a breast cancer diagnosis in her lifetime.

- Breast cancer is typically diagnosed in women, even though men are also susceptible. However rare, an average of 2,470 males will get breast cancer annually, and 460 will succumb to the disease each year.

- Breast Cancer is the leading cause of death for women. Every 2 minutes, a woman is diagnosed and will die every 13 minutes.

- There are an estimated 13.3 million breast cancer survivors in this country.

Genes matter.

A hereditary cancer gene is when a person is a carrier of a cell mutation gene that can transfer from parent to child. Most often, people want to find out if this applies to them for prevention reasons and to save their own lives in catching cancer early and developing treatment and prevention plans. A genetic counselor and doctor will more than likely provide detailed information to a patient on what this all involves.

This, in essence, means that you have had a test conducted by a medical professional that has identified you as a possible candidate for hereditary cancer. The only way to determine this fact is through a bonafide genetic test involving sampling saliva or blood and sending it to a laboratory for testing.

This was different than any test available when my mother was alive. It took just a minute to perform this on myself and each of my children. Unfortunately, after it was all said and done, the nurse informed me that the test was inconclusive.

So, am I right back where I started?

America is a melting pot of cultures and ethnicities. The byproduct of that produced diverse family components incorporating those various nationalities. This reality can sometimes make it challenging to learn if genetic testing is necessary.

The easier way to do this is to simply ask family and extended family members if they are aware of or have any knowledge of members of the family who had acquired cancer? This knowledge represents the power to take control of your health.

Education matters.

Being educated and aware of breast cancer, genetically linked or not, will decrease the rise in mortality rates involving this disease.

In my case, I had to inquire from my grandparents and parents on my dad's side of the family to come up with a reasonable amount of information that would give me just cause to have the test conducted.

Because of the stigma that can sometimes surround this disease, it became difficult to gather much of this information.

I decided to have the genetic testing done since I was a mother, and I wanted to equip my children with vital information just in case it could save their lives.

I finally realized why people weren't forthcoming with this information. It was about shame. They would be breaking the golden rule of family privacy. "What happens in this house stays in this house."

Science matters.

Let me explain some details so you can gain a clearer picture. A gene is made up of the DNA from each cell inside your body. Genes predict how cells grow, divide, and their length of life.

Scientific experts state that there are at least 30,000 various genes in each cell. Inside each cell, the genes are house by chromosomes. Chromosomes look like small threads connecting cells to genes.

Every living person obtains a single set of chromosomes from their mother and a single set from their father.

These chromosomes predict if you will be male or female and other physical attributes.

This is how genes operate. Collectively the chromosomes are known as autosomes. Genes help cells produce proteins. Proteins send messages to cells.

Cancer cells start when one or more cells start to mutate. This creates a change in the cell's composition and functioning. An abnormal protein sends a different message than a normal one. This causes cells to grow uncontrollably and turn into cancer.

There are two types of genetic mutations:

- Acquired mutations, where there is damage done to the gene throughout an individual's life where cells began to multiply and create a tumor. Elements that may cause these mutations are tobacco, ultraviolet radiation, viruses, and age. Acquired mutations are not inherited.

- Germline mutations happen in sperm or egg cells and are inherited from parent to child at conception. When the embryo turns into a baby, these mutations are duplicated in every cell in the body. This mutation impacts the reproductive system and passes within generations. These cancers spread by germline mutations are typically known as inherited cancers. It collectively makes up between 5-20 percent of all known cancers.

If we were to dig a little deeper into this, mutations occur quite often and can be good and bad. It all depends on the actual change.

The body automatically takes care of incorrect mutations. One mutation will not cause cancer. It is when these mutations occur over a lifetime and build up that cancer can take place.

These are the types of genes linked to cancer:

- Tumor suppressor genes are usually protective. They often cease cell development by overseeing when cells grow and divide, repair DNA, and when cells die. Tumor suppressor genes can cause cells to grow uncontrollably and turn into a tumor.

  For example, tumor suppressor genes are BRAC1, BRAC2, and p53, TP53. Germline mutations found in BRAC1 and BRAC2 can increase a women's risk of getting hereditary breast cancer and prostate or breast cancer for men. People with the p53 and TP53 gene mutations are at a higher risk of developing acquired cancer.

- Another is called Oncogenes, which are healthy cells that turn cancerous and are not inherited. Typical oncogenes are HER2, a protein that controls how cancers grow and spread.

- RAS is a collection of genes where proteins communicate messages to the life or death of a cell.

Oncology researchers continue to learn more about what makes these genes operate. But unfortunately, many cancers are not connected to a particular gene. More than likely, it is connected to several forms of gene mutations. Improvements in this area include cancer care, early detection, and targeted therapy.

Tests matter.

There are several different types of genetic tests. There are tests that concentrate on a designated area of a single gene and its mutation, while others study one gene searching for any signs of mutation

Other genetic tests are known as panel tests that analyze a collection of genes for mutations at the same time. These tests combine 5 or 6 genes and even up to 30 genes for next-generation gene sequencing. These are tests that use the latest technology to look for the sequence patterns in several genes.

These particular tests search for BRCA1 or BRCA2 mutations in addition to inherited mutations connected to breast cancer risk like:

ATM	BRIP1	CDH1
CHEK2	MRE11A	MSH6
NBN	p53	PALB2
PTEN	RAD50	RAD51C
STK11	TP53	

A genetic practitioner or doctor can assist with answering questions about the various options available.

Discovery matters.

Cancer that is passed from parent to child is called hereditary cancer syndrome. This is a specific form of inherited conditions where an increased risk of developing certain types of cancer is possible.

Hereditary Cancer Syndrome is usually passed to the child by the parent. This transmission is quite often apparent within families. This would include a sister, mother, or daughter who has developed cancer or acquired cancer at an early age. Ovarian and breast cancer are both connected to heredity cancer syndrome.

My initial encounter with genetic tests came by way of my oncologist. I had children, and the physician thought I would want to know if I was a carrier of the cancer gene. My children were also tested.

Genetic testing seeks changes in an individual's genes or variants. These can be harmful or beneficial to the risk of the development of cancer. Inherited variants are believed to be a major contributor in 5-10 percent to most of the cancers. It may seem as if cancer "runs in families" even when this variant is not the cause. Tobacco, alcohol, and shared lifestyle may cause a similar development of certain cancers.

Particular types of genes are suspected to be part of inherited cancer susceptibility syndrome. Deciding to test to determine if someone is a carrier of a harmful variant in genes would confirm its validity. Genetic testing is also useful in determining if a family member has inherited this variant.

There is also a different type of genetic testing called tumor DNA sequencing, which is performed to see if any cells or genetic changes are identified that can be helpful for treatment.

Inheriting the cancer susceptibility doesn't always mean you will get cancer. If the cancer susceptibility in a part of your family dynamics, other factors can determine the onset of the disease.

The main factor influencing whether a person acquires this disease is what's called a variance penetrance. This means some people may get the disease while others may not. This is called incomplete or reduced penetrance.

People with hereditary cancer syndrome can have the disease with various expressivity, meaning it could or could not show physical signs or symptoms. Lifestyle and environmental factors are predicted to influence the disease.

People have several reasons for getting genetic testing. Your physician may feel it may be a good idea for patients with children or other family members may have or had the disease. The test is totally voluntary.

A counselor usually aids in helping families consider the benefits of the test. These professionals assist in the understanding of the scientific, emotional, and ethical components of the decision to test or not and its results.

Counseling and testing are usually recommended for those people with a pattern of cancers. The following could be good reasons to get tested:

- First degree relatives like mother, father, sisters, brothers, or children who have had cancer.

- Relatives on either side of the family who were diagnosed with a similar kind of cancer such as breast, ovarian, and pancreatic cancers.

- Members who have had several types of cancer.

- Members who acquired cancer at a young age.

- Relatives who had cancer connected to hereditary cancer syndrome.

Diagnostic tests are typically recommended to detect any diseases which could cause illness in a person. The conclusion of such a test will aid in making decisions on health management.

Analyzing the changes in genes helps to determine a link in the onset of the disease. The outcome of these tests gives information on risk levels for diseases such as breast cancer.

In addition, carrier testing is conducted on people who are suspected carriers of the gene connected to a disease. While a carrier may not show any symptoms of the abnormal gene mutation, they can still pass it on to their children.

Genetic counseling matters.

Current studies show that genetic testing plays a role in finding out gene functioning as a benefit or harm to the body.

There is an excess of 50 hereditary cancer syndromes.

Individuals who have a concern about if their family history places them at risk for cancer or breast cancer should speak with a doctor about genetic testing.

Also, an individual's family history may place them at risk of hereditary cancer syndrome.

This is what to look out for:

- An early cancer diagnosis.

- Various types of cancer happened in one person.

- Cancer detected in other organs like both kidneys and both breasts.

- Finding out your risk can help prevent future cancer.

- Family members who are carriers of the inherited genetic variant.

When a person is subject to having inherited cancer susceptibility syndrome, one or more family members have the variant recommended that they have genetic testing.

Remember that early detection saves lives.

Genetic counseling usually takes place before a genetic test is conducted for signs of hereditary cancer syndrome.

When a person has a positive result, and they do, in fact, have the syndrome, then the composition of the cells is analyzed further to gain more specific information.

This information is used to formulate a precancerous plan that would include future testing and any prerequisites to treating these risk factors.

A trained counselor and health care professional will then take the necessary action. This will include:

- A risk assessment considering family medical history.

- A conversation about the pros and cons of genetic testing.

- Testing results could be positive, negative, or inconclusive.

- The possibility of passing the variants to children.

- What the genetic test means to the family involved.

- The specific recommended test to perform.

- Support groups for the patient.

- Test benefits and risks.

- The genetic test shows data about the patient and the family.

Genetic testing is typically requested by the patient's doctor or other health care professional. They would analyze a single gene or a harmful variant in a collection of genes.

A small bodily fluid sample or tissue like blood, saliva, or skin. This sample is sent to a laboratory for genetic testing. Results from the test usually take about 2 weeks. Insurance will usually cover the cost of the test if the doctor deems it necessary.

Results from genetic testing could determine what current cancers are attributed to an inherited genetic variant. This could also mean identifying additional risk for acquiring particular cancers in the future and assist with managing these risks.

Genetic counselors will provide additional information to assist the patient and family members as they decide their health care options available to them and ways to lower risks in finding cancer early. A negative result could mean that the patient does not have inherited cancer susceptibility syndrome.

Overall, information matters. It's always good to educate yourself in any way you can.

You should explore your family history, your genetic makeup, and all research on tests and scientific information that you can get your hands on.

Somewhere in the midst of my haste, I was informed that my insurance had lapsed. Fixing this dilemma was easier said than done.

It took a great deal of legwork until the patient advocate at the oncologist's office stepped in and pulled together her known resources and enrolled me in a program that would take care of all the cancer-related and other medical expenses.

This same advocate put me in touch with organizations that help to pay rent, utility bills, and other household and living expenses. This was a godsend. The comfort of knowing that I was not the only person looking for financial assistance was a comfort to my family and me.

One of the most emotionally draining experiences for me is the possibility that cancer may return and be able to finance my health care and living expenses. When undergoing treatment for breast cancer, it is helpful always to have as many options available to you in case you need to call on them for help.

There were many instances where I had to research available resources that would cover medication, items not covered by traditional insurance, and monetary supplements for missed days of work. See Appendix C for a listing of organizations that may be able to offer financial assistance.

I had to make a tough decision. Could I keep my job and my independence?

Legal matters.

My supervisors knew what was going on with my health and that I wanted to continue to be employed. This would sometimes mean some missed days and work hours to get treatment, tests, and overall check-ups.

I was hopeful that they would understand and not find a replacement for my position. These are some of the concerns patients would more than likely concern themselves with, especially those with children without partners to pitch in.

Currently, there are three federal laws that protect employees with a long-term illness such as cancer. These regulations are called the EEOC or Equal Employment Opportunities Commission.

The Americans with Disabilities Act or ADA protects employees from negative employment action based on their disability. Employers must also make reasonable accommodations for the disability.

The Genetic Information Nondiscrimination Act (GINA) says that genetic testing and information cannot be requested by employers or health insurers. Your genetic testing remains private.

The Family Medical Leave Act (FMLA) gives employees up to 12 weeks of job-protected unpaid leave. This helps eligible employees keep their jobs and from employers retaliating against taking time off for eligible circumstances.

Credentials matter.

I can recall this particular instance where my mother had begun to seek this soothsayer or doctor-of-sorts who promised to work miracles in the area of healing cancer and other life-threatening illnesses. He even had witnesses to testify that he was legit.

In my mother's rush to cure her cancer, she had depleted all of her savings on paying this healer. This is something to be aware of - people who claim to work miracles. I'll be the first one to tell you that I am a firm believer in miracles, but we have to look at the bigger picture.

Rely on the doctors with credentials you can readily check on and even then get a second opinion. My family had mobilized at our house and promised to give all they could to help pay for this alternative therapy.

I am not saying this person was a thief, he very well could have had some proven miracles under his belt. But be careful.

Spending everything you have on a "wing and a prayer" in hopes of being cancer-free means taking a huge chance on something and someone that may be a scammer.

I have always believed that people prey on desperation. This is very similar to those "get-rich-quick schemes."

Let's take a look at this for a moment. If someone had the ultimate cure for diseases, why didn't everybody have access to this knowledge? Why was the cost so expensive for the average person to afford? And why did they operate their practice in such secrecy?

As I mentioned before, some people live and breathe on signs and wonders. All I am saying is to be practical.

Your best bet is consulting a reputable doctor with an actual Ph.D. A few of the top cancer hospitals in the nation are:

- University of Texas MD Anderson Cancer Center in Houston

- Memorial Sloan Kettering Cancer Center in Houston

- Mayo Clinic in Rochester

- Birmingham and Women's Hospital in Boston

- Dana-Farber Cancer Institute in Boston

- UCLA Medical Center in Los Angeles

- Moffitt Cancer Center and Research Institute in Tampa

- University of Washington Medical Center in Seattle

- Seattle Center Care Alliance in Seattle

- Cleveland Clinic in Cleveland

Coworker matters.

My experience at work with coworkers, staff, my boss, and others seemed as if they were walking on eggshells or tiptoeing around me constantly inquiring as to how I am feeling.

I felt ostracized in their efforts to be inclusive of me. I saw the stares when they felt I wasn't paying attention.

Despite the illness, I was still a force to be reckoned with. People seemed to feel that you couldn't have a regular conversation or dialogue devoid of cancer.

Initial situations relied on successfully getting through the day.

People needed to learn cancer survivors were regular individuals and didn't want special attention for a normal day's work.

Don't talk to me like I am a little child.

I am an adult capable of an adult conversation, I thought to myself. The tone of their voice changes, their body demeanor changes to accommodate your presence.

An employee raised her voice at me, laced in venom. I stood up and yelled back. I could hold my own.

I may be a survivor, but I was certainly not a pushover or a sucker. Bring it.

Once the tirades were over, as we stood toe to toe in the workplace, the other staff members began to recognize that I was a regular person. They would have never known I had cancer based on my actions and attitude.

That's just the effect I wanted to make. Cancer did not make me weak.

My supervisors were very understanding when I revealed I had a cancer diagnosis and that it required intense treatment, therapy, and surgery.

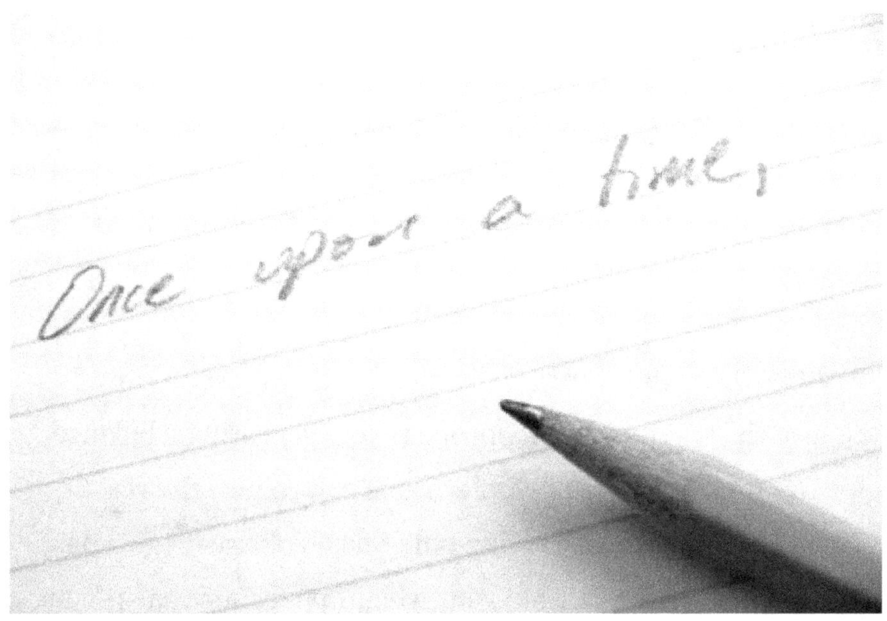

There are several popular myths and misconceptions surrounding how a person develops breast cancer.

Some of those notions include the use of aerosol deodorants, wearing bras that contain underwire, and certain body soaps will cause breast cancer. All of these are wrong.

Myth: Women with small breasts are the least at risk for developing breast cancer than those with larger breasts.

Truth: Women of all sizes can be subject to developing breast cancer.

Myth: Breast cancer is for women only.

Truth: Men are also diagnosed with breast cancer.

Myth: There is nothing a person can do to prevent breast cancer.

Truth: Quite the contrary, living a healthy lifestyle can reduce risks. For example, proper exercise, eating a balanced, low-fat diet inclusive of whole grains can reduce the risk of getting breast cancer. Having only one alcoholic drink a day, no smoking, and watching your weight post-menopause can also help to diminish to chances of developing breast cancer.

Myth: A biopsy makes cancer spread.

Truth: There is absolutely no truth that having a biopsy or mammogram causes any cancers to spread.

Myth: A patient diagnosed with cancer should have surgery immediately.

Truth: The reality is that a patient who has been diagnosed with cancer should wait and get a second doctor's opinion before deciding the next course of action – surgery or not.

<u>Myth:</u> Having a lumpectomy instead of mastectomy increases the life expectancy for cancer patients.

Truth: The life expectancy is about the same amount for either procedure.

<u>Myth:</u> Only people with a family history of cancer are at risk for developing breast cancer.

Truth: The truth is that 80 percent of cancer patients do not have a family history of breast cancer or any other kind of cancer.

More Truth: Of the 12 percent of women who develop breast cancer in their lifetime, only 55-65 percent get it from the harmful, inherited BRCA1 or BRCA2 mutation.

Even More Truth: The risk of breast cancer increases with age. It is recommended that women aged 70 and beyond continue to get their yearly mammograms.

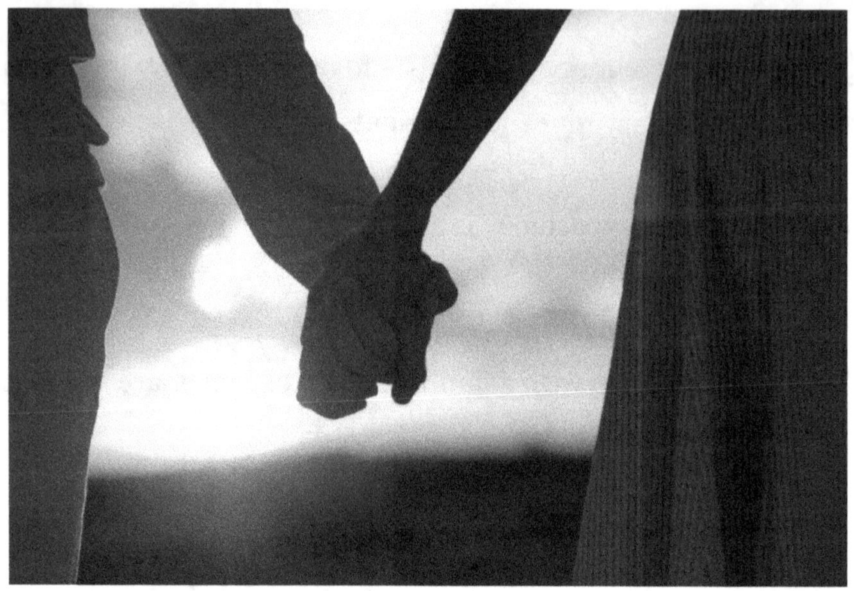

I thought of my best friend, Gloria. I hadn't spoken to her in over 10 years, and nonetheless, she was the first person I thought about sharing this news with outside of my immediate family.

We had some squabble about something I can't even recall that created the distance which emerged between us.

We used to talk about everything, I do mean everything. Some things we would surely take to the grave.

I had passed by her house a thousand times over that time. I showed up at her door. And she came and reached out her arms and said, "What's wrong?"

It was a rainy and chilly morning when I met Gloria. She was driving and passed by me with the kids walking to their schools. My car was down for the count, and the kids and I hoovered together briskly on the path.

Gloria blew her horn, "Where you on the way to? Get in!" I hesitated, as did the kids.

I guess they thought surely mom is not going to get in the car with a stranger. This was totally against the rules.

Gloria continued to implore us to take a ride with her to the school. We did ultimately, and we chit-chatted once the kids were dropped off. I told her where we lived, and she told me likewise.

There was another incident where we crossed paths again. Before you knew it, we were meeting and gathering often and began to share secrets about our lives. Two years in, I got a divorce, Gloria remained with her suitor, found out he was cheating and took him back.

We were both motherless, and I guess that is the main fact that drew us together.

We became the financial, emotional, and psychological anchors for one another. We had mad parties, and both felt rejuvenated in each other's company.

We were best friends.

Best friends matter.

We had dinners at her house. One of the main things that stood out over the course of the friendship is the delicious meals she would prepare in our honor.

On one of those dinner nights, I had invited a guest, and there was something said which rubbed Gloria the wrong way, and heated words were exchanged. I cannot even recall the exact words that were said.

This blew way out of proportion, and we stopped talking. Neither one of us felt the other was in the wrong, and neither one of us were going to make the first move to squash the beef.

Soon, distance had come between us. One day turned into months. Months turned into years.

When I approached her door, I didn't know what to expect. The cancer survival had given me new-found courage to conquer anything, especially fear of the unknown.

Besides hello, I told her about the information that I had acquired cancer. She dropped to the floor in anguish. We cried together, brushed ourselves off, and prepared for the next game plan.

She was very supportive as usual and became as expected – additional ammunition in overcoming the disease with ease. She was the shoulder I never felt I needed and the wings to keep me moving in the right direction.

Before that day, ongoing conversations would stop when I entered the room with those who were aware of my condition. I was a stranger in their midst.

I think this attitude from others stemmed from not being educated or aware of breast cancer and those who had been diagnosed with the disease. It was an unfamiliar ground for many. It could be fear in knowing they could get the disease also. This is where the myths arise, grow, and fester.

Gloria and I sat on the porch in the rocking chair sofa, rocking back and forth, catching up on lost time, things that happened in our absence, and the people and events that made us giggle endlessly through the evening.

We stopped the movements from time to time to emphasize different points to our stories by slapping our knees, only to laugh some more.

These were the good old times I remembered. She was just as I recalled, the same study rock that I depended on.

I had always heard some people come into your life for a season to give support, knowledge to bring peace, comfort or a much-needed spiritual message of comfort. But I had changed. I no longer lived by the seat of my britches. My decisions were more calculated and well-thought-out.

Moving on matters.

It wasn't that I couldn't remember the joys and the spices of life or the feel of the closeness of another next to me. I didn't want to. I was unwilling to become too comfortable, only to have the rug pulled right out from under me and forget all about the slippery slope that I stood upon.

That lying, stinking, filthy, cunning foundation that coerced me into thinking the world was mine to do with it as I pleased.

I wasn't going to set myself up for an excruciating and painful downfall this time.

The cancer had taught me not to depend on anything or anyone - that nothing was for certain or held any assuredness.

Still, I missed those days. I longed for the old me. The one who challenged the mountains that stood in my way of progress.

I twirled my thumbs together, waiting for a sign. I needed permission or a go-ahead from this elusive force that has held me captive and controlled my every step.

I was always taught to have a Plan B. In this way, the disappointments won't destroy you, and you can soon rise again on a new path. I should have known better.

I didn't want to delve too deep into this line of reasoning to the point of no return.

I had more important things to consider, like how to face an uncertain future without a hitch.

I needed to realize how not to go after those things in life that I had once craved, which were now beyond my reach.

I've always suffered from violent nightmares my whole life. Far from the kind where you wake up out of a deep sleep in a cold sweat, but the kind where someone or something was always chasing me all the way to the end of a cliff and I could either jump into the air over it to my demise or fight my way through the attacker. Loud screams would erupt.

To me, the dreams were real. Shaking me out of the dreamlike state could be dangerous. I was fighting for my life in each dream.

I remember this callous doctor telling me that sometimes nightmares come true, referring to my mother and her cancer diagnosis. I never forgot the abrasive manner in which he delivered the message. And now, I was faced with delivering this same message to my children, only with kindness and love.

Some memories are simply too painful to recall. While these events are long past, they leave unshakable residue on the psyche. The body doesn't control the mind, the mind controls the body.

I felt faint from the preview of recounting these words to the kids. Besides hearing the shocking news from my doctor stating I had cancer, I felt like I was walking down a primrose path. In other words, I was taking a journey to meet my maker finally. I remember reading that word in a novel some time ago and never imagined what it meant. Now I know.

At one of the children's school meetings, I went in, greeted everyone, and sat down to have the conference with my child's teacher.

I could tell the way she held her head to the side, leaning forward, she knew I had cancer. My daughter had told her.

I kept telling myself, even through this experience, there is a difference between being empathetic and understanding another one's condition or circumstances and quite another to feel sad for the person.

There is a distinct line between feeling sorry for a person and genuinely being remorseful and pitying them.

Giving in to the latter could be catastrophic to my state of mind and future well-being. I tried to the best of my ability to act normal. Whatever that means.

There's a difference between pity and concern. Pity can be very destructive.

Case in point: I was walking, and I accidentally tripped over something in my path, and I stumbled. Everyone turned around, gasping in alarm. When I said I was fine, and it was just a minor fluke, I looked at them as they stared at me. They didn't know what to say or what to do. I assured them everything was okay. I had this sinking feeling they weren't convinced from the trembling of my voice.

Have you ever experienced something like a loss of a loved one or dear friend, or lost a long-term job where everything you have worked for your whole life goes up in smoke? Once the news broke out about it, you were so traumatized you couldn't even cry about it? Where I come from, crying meant defeat, and I wasn't giving up just yet.

My son seemed to carry the burden the most. I knew him. I was his mother, and I knew when something deep down was weighing heavily on his heart.

When he came home from school one day, I had his favorite song playing and grabbed his hand and said, "Dance with me."

His reaction was silence combined with a look on his face as if I had just lost my mind.

We shimmed around singing the words to the song out loud and pretended to go back in time to when I taught him how to swing dance. That's what old people do, you know, they do dances like no one's watching.

After some time of doing this, we just looked at each other and laughed. It was a long time since we laughed together. Things had become so serious, we forgot about some of the finer aspects of life. The little things that made life worth living.

The next day, I knew I had to brace myself. I just wanted to ask everyone who looked at me funny, "Why are you staring at me like you were expecting death to walk through the door?"

I am still the same person, I merely have to overcome this bump in the road, and things will ultimately continue as normal. The problem is, I didn't feel like I used to.

Something had changed, and things would never be as they once were. Not in a bad or negative sense but rather just that things had changed.

I was deep down inside not the same person.

I pretended to be a runway model, stopping here and there to strike a pose, then twisting and turning to ensure that the audience received a full view. This was all played out in my head.

Let me back up. After my conversation with the children as a group, I spoke to each one of them directly and asked them to tell me how they were feeling and coping with the cancer news.

Each asked if there was hope for a cure, and the doctors were actively working on making the experience a thing of the past. They were on board with the whole matter. I took a chance and gave them specific information and details, which I thought they could handle and not too much which could potentially generate fear.

I worked diligently to create a sense of normalcy in the home. I continued to work, plan outings, and secure a future with me in it.

My attitude and mood would set the tone for a home filled with love, security, and hope. Besides a strong sense of loss, the children would feel if something were to happen to me, there was equally a strong sense of insecurity that clouded each day.

In the next chapter, I will discuss more in length about how to approach the cancer conversation with children.

57

Children Matter

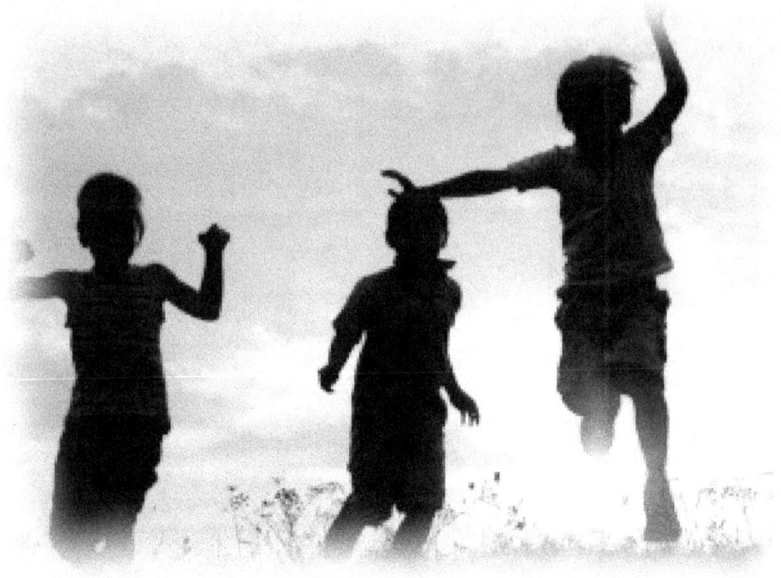

Looking at the children hanging on my every word, I had to leave some information out when I finally told them about the severity of my illness.

The youngest one's first words were, "Will I get it too and die?"

Boy, oh boy, my theatre minor in college was sure to come in handy now!

I was not ready for the question. I had prepared myself for questions like, "Where do babies come from? What is sex? Why can't I spend the night with my friend? Are you getting a divorce from dad? Will we be poor?"

I could handle those questions with some level of authenticity and finesse. Yet, how could I answer a question where I didn't control the outcome?

I dug deep. I replied, "Of course not, honey. Why would you think of such a thing?"

I knew all the while why the question was asked. I wanted to ask the medical team the same damn thing.

Who in the world wants to answer a question like this to someone who hasn't gone on their first date, experienced their first crush, had their first kiss, or went to college away from home?

This was going to be a long one. I said it as calmly and matter-of-factly as if it didn't stumble me in the least bit. They each peered at me as they had done in the past as if my answers to their questions were written in stone and I sat next to Jesus, almighty.

The times in their lives where I answered their questions with, "I don't know, honey," were few and far between. I wanted to keep it that way.

I hypothetically looked up the best practices on explaining death to a child, just in case I had to equip myself with an arsenal. Fortunately, I haven't had to resort to this, thank goodness.

The children seemed puzzled, satisfied with my responses, yet still perplexed. How do I tackle wiping that look off their faces?

The family slept uneasily that night. The little one came into my room and bowled herself into a cocoon under my arm like she needed me to shield her for what would come next.

The delivery matters.

This is how I approached the challenge earlier that evening.

I sat upright, straight in the chair, and told them I was diagnosed with breast cancer and would need to undergo treatment to kill the cancer cells in my body to live. I explained what this would involve having surgery to remove the bad cancer cells in my body, then taking preventive medicine, radiation therapy, and chemotherapy that would make me lose my hair and potentially cause me to feel sick to my stomach for a short time.

I'd said a mouthful. Each of them was filled with questions that I answered to the best of my ability.

Mostly, they wanted to return to the innocent state they were in before I uttered a word.

Without being too technical, I broke down the information about cancer and stopped each time they had questions.

They cried ferociously, and the following day, they went about their daily duties, carrying around this information lodged in their minds.

My son accompanied me to every treatment session, and we made small talk about the news, TV shows, movies that were coming out, and which ones we would go see together.

I didn't feel hopeful, although I had to pretend everything was going to be alright.

You know how the old saying goes, "Fake it till you make it."

I wondered if the children deserved to hear this from someone who had always taken care of every hurdle in their lives since they were young.

I weaved in the truth and dispelled the myths surrounding the disease to them so they would know the real deal, straight from the horse's mouth, so to speak. We bought books that helped to reinforce the information. Whatever was going to help them reach some peace with this knowledge, we explored.

Each doctor on the medical team agreed to schedule a meeting with the children on one of my visits. They provided more details to the questions asked and assured them they had caught the cancer early, which increased my survival rate.

Each professional answered the children's' questions thoroughly, showed visuals, and gave them comfort by making them a part of this experience. They took packets home to review and refer to in case there were further questions and concerns.

Contact numbers were given out to the children with an open invitation to call at any time. This was a big deal and made the children feel like they were not being kept in the dark about such an important and critical matter.

As we drove away from the doctor's offices, I could hear the sighs of relief coming from the backseat. They were sad but empowered and hopeful.

Normalcy matters.

Slowly, but surely the kids began to come around from the devastating news, and I started to look more and more like the mother they'd always known. After one of the doctor's visits, my daughter and I sat on the bench outside, and she looked so serious - not like the carefree, innocent young girl I'd hoped she'd become.

Spontaneously, I picked up one of the green, stalk-shaped plants with a white, soft pointed top growing in the grass where we sat and blew it towards her. It looked like a mini snowstorm. She looked at me, aghast. Her face spoke volumes. Her look was, "Don't you know we are dealing with something serious here?"

I would blow the furballs towards her all the time when she was a little girl, and she would laugh hysterically, blowing them back at me. It was a happy, joyous time back then.

I know they were scared. Scared of the unknown. Sometimes, even as adults, fear of the unknown can take on a life of its own. A living, breathing, intangible thing that grows uncontrollably until our thoughts stop feeding into it.

As I went about being the mother they remembered, I would catch them staring at me from time to time. I could only wonder what they could be thinking.

Since I wasn't walking around, humped over with a walking cane as most people literally believed, and they had imagined. I did the same things every day I used to do, like going to their schools, taking them to work, getting school supplies, shopping for an upcoming event for them, celebrated birthdays, and planned outings.

I could see in their eyes that they were reassured things would work out fine after all.

Strategies matter.

Most people who have experienced a cancer diagnosis worry about how the illness and treatment will impact their families. They also tend to be very concerned about how to tell their children about cancer.

There are some clear-cut strategies for communicating with children about cancer.

How much information should a family member share with the children regarding a cancer diagnosis? A good rule of thumb from my experience is to refrain from revealing anything that may cause fear or discomfort. Tell the truth of the severity of the issue, but reassure the children that they are not the cause of the situation.

Talking to children about a cancer diagnosis is not easy. But honesty is the best policy. Open discussions on the topic make children feel less afraid and allow them to express their feelings on the matter.

It is best to talk to children soon after the cancer diagnosis. Talking about the issue of early aids in building trust by keeping them in the loop.

Before you talk to the children, prepare for the conversation. Practice or write down the important points to the conversation. Decide what you want to say and how much you want to say makes things easier and a little less stressful.

Find a quiet space in which to hold the conversation, away from any distractions that may arise. The conversation is difficult enough, let alone with constant interruptions. Host this conversation at the quietest time of the day when children are not busy and can be relaxed.

For children of different ages, it is best to tell each child individually close to the same time. This will allow each child the opportunity to support each other. Be as understanding as possible, letting them know you are aware of how they must be feeling.

This is another caveat. What you have to say is just as important as how you say it. Try to be as understanding as possible, even if one or more of the children walk away from the conversation. Let them know that it is okay to cry and express whatever they may feel at the time.

When and if children ask questions that you may not be sure about, let them know that you will find out the answer as soon as possible.

Children typically have a short attention span, so don't push too much information on them at the same time. Gradually divulge the necessary and needed important information.

Don't use language and words that the child may not be familiar with. Break it down to them in small chunks of information a little at a time. Explain things on their developmental level so that they can understand about what cancer is and what to look for days ahead.

Find out what the child may have heard about cancer in order to clear up any misconceptions. Be sure to listen as well as share any additional necessary details. Let them know that it is okay to ask any questions they may have regarding the situation.

Reassure small children that they did not do anything to cause the sickness, and it is not their fault. Be sure also to let them know that cancer is not the kind of illness that is contagious like a cold.

It is not uncommon for parents to feel unsure and uneasy about sharing this information with their kids. Just letting them know at the outset that you are there for them no matter what is helpful to ease any fears they may have.

There aren't any right or wrong ways to have this conversation with children. Keeping conversations about the cancer diagnosis simple and open works best in making them feel secure and hopeful.

Reinforce to the children that it is okay to ask any questions they what answers to and that you are always available to them to talk about their concerns. This may be the first of many conversations down the road.

Determine who you wish to be present when you break the news to the children for support. It could be a friend, family, or clergy member. These agents can help soften the blow about the cancer news and reassure the children they are available to help.

Prepare yourself for the dreaded question from the children of "Are you going to die?" Be honest with the children and explain that some people do die from the disease but that many live and recover from the illness successfully. Explain to children that the doctors are working hard to get rid of all cancer from your body so that you can live a long, healthy life.

Allow the children time to take in the cancer news. Many children express themselves and how they are feeling through their behaviors.

Some are verbal, but many show their true feelings through their actions. Parents need to be patient with the children as they go through this struggle of absorbing the news.

As the surgery date drew closer, I decided to have a sit down with my eldest child about my end of life plan. I felt he was old enough to handle the conversation.

The administrators had given me paperwork in the preop office about the end of life procedure or protocol. I completed the paperwork and now had to have the talk with my child.

I explained to him where the insurance papers were kept, how I wish things to be implemented, like taking care of his siblings. I told him how I didn't want resuscitation if something were to occur on the operating table. He wasn't pleased, yet he agreed to follow through with my requests.

I guess, in the living and surviving, not living or not surviving never really came up in any previous conversations. Now was the time to put everything in order.

I went over every inch of the paperwork with him, how I wanted the insurance money distributed and where I wanted my belongings to go.

This conversation really put the big picture into perspective.

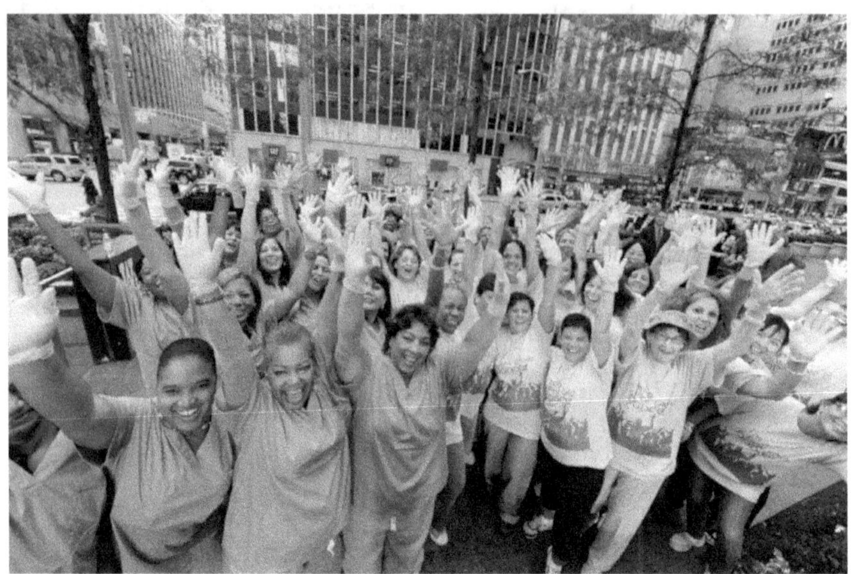

On operation day, we drove to the hospital in complete silence. When we arrived at the facility, I went into a room, then waited to go into another room to prepare for the actual operation.

Nurses started an IV, and the surgeon came to check to see how I was fairing. I really didn't know what to expect. It's not like I had anything else to compare it to.

I decided to have a mastectomy to remove the cancer from my body. I had already seen the visuals and the pictures when I met with this physician. She had explained every inch of what would take place and wanted to ensure I understood how the procedure would go and what it would entail.

Earlier on in my cancer journey, my oncologist told me I had the BRCA2. There is also a BRACA1. These genes contain what is called suppressor proteins.

The job of these proteins is to heal damaged DNA to reinforce the ability of a cell's genetic make-up to function properly. Regardless if the gene mutation is changed or whether the protein is developed or doesn't operate correctly, damage to the DNA may not be repaired correctly. Thus, cells will create more genetic alterations, which may cause cancer.

Certain mutations inherited in BRAC1 and BRAC2 increase the onset of breast cancer and other types of cancers. Dangerous BRCA1 and BRAC2 may be inherited from either the mother or the father. Experts contend that parents who are carriers of the harmful BRAC1 and BRAC2 mutations have a 50% chance of passing on the mutation.

This is the foundation for cancer risk management, which may include surveillance, often checking to see if there are any changes to your body, screenings by taking mammograms and

MRIs with the focus to catch any signs of cancer at its early stages.

The most common breast cancer risk reduction strategies are mastectomy with breast reconstruction afterward. This is the surgery I had performed on me. This type of operation is recommended to reduce breast cancer risk and its reoccurrence.

Breast cancer risk is higher between the ages of 30-60. A person's overall health condition plays a vital role in the impact of these risks.

Oncologists highly recommend risk-reducing surgery for those people who are identified as carriers of BRCA1 or BRCA2 mutations. Identifying hereditary BRAC1 or BRAC2 during the initial testing of a person with cancer is beneficial because it allows for early treatment and access to more therapies.

Being proactive matters.

It's important to take an active part in your breast cancer treatment and healing. Take notes or prepare questions to ask the medical team. Reach a greater understanding of the process and what's involved in your healing.

In my experience, breast cancer survivors tend to do one of several things. They avoid the discussion altogether because it is a constant reminder of coming face to face with their own mortality. They live their cancer condition overzealously, meaning everything and everybody and their entire being is centered around cancer where they forget to live aside from it. They approach life in denial like nothing ever happened.

Each one of these reactions to a breast cancer diagnosis could be detrimental to the person's well-being. Survivors can either choose to have the disease consume them or accept the reality of their condition, taking an active role in their lives.

Breast cancer can be a harrowing, nail-biting experience, although doing your homework and finding out new therapies, available clinical trials, and staying abreast of the latest developments on the subject can give you just the confidence required to get through this journey successfully.

In my case, the psychological aspect attached to the disease was more trying than the disease itself. Considering that my mother had died of the very thing I have now been diagnosed with significantly reduced my positive attitude towards the medical team.

We had several conferences and hours upon hours of discussions on the matter at hand. It took some time for me to come around and accept the fact that I had acquired the disease, and it was inherited. Why couldn't I have just gotten hazel eyes, fair skin, and a knock-out body from my parents?

When I speak of cancer, I remembered the bad days my mother would struggle through with the disease tagging along right behind her. The sickness and lack of energy where she could barely get out of bed was heartbreaking. The desire to endure this torture was not an appealing one for me.

I had to change the narrative about breast cancer survivors.

To say this experience has changed my life is an understatement. Things I'd previously said no to, I considered. I began to become vocal. I became more visible in cancer circles and raised money for those patients who were challenged financially with obtaining adequate healthcare.

I read continuously about triumphant survivor stories and the elements which helped these survivors on the bad days.

I began to approach life with a sense of newness and vigor. I surrounded myself with the goodness of life while being a participant in life and not just an innocent bystander on the outside looking in.

Put one foot in front of the other.

This is a simple command that will carry you a long way on your path. An essential key element to surviving this experience is to bring balance to your life aside from the cancer activities.

I learned to salsa dance. The moves were so intoxicating, and the music drew me closer to my soul.

I became fearless and fierce. I started writing down my feelings in a journal. Writing became my therapeutic expression.

The takeaway from this is making peace with the situation. Once this is accomplished, you are well on your way to creating your new normal, including dismantling limitless barriers that had hindered you prior to the cancer diagnosis.

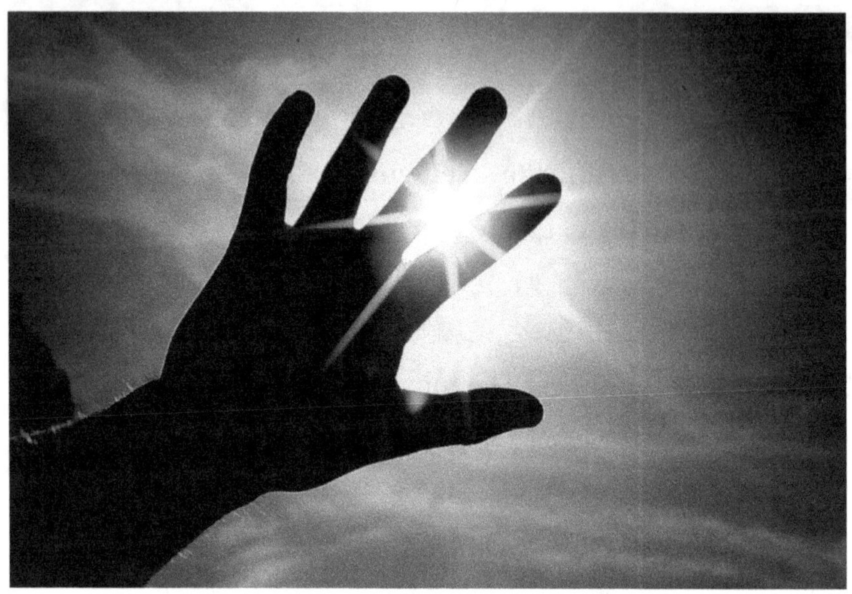

Having survived breast cancer and its aftermath, I was increasingly concerned with methods to grow my hair back and increase my energy level.

In my empowerment, I came across a few ideas. I started taking multivitamins and eating three healthy meals a day. I also started taking biotin supplements since I'd heard it helps to stimulate hair follicles. There was some improvement, but simply doing something about my condition aided in my mental state on the issue.

I read the pamphlet in the doctor's office, talked to the patient advocate, and found out about the different activities available to survivors. The initial plans to salsa dance became too exhausting. Perhaps I can try again later down the line in my recovery.

I selected the yoga option instead. It was the most peaceful experience I had in a long time. The meditation aspect of the exercise was the best. I joined a group with other survivors, and it gave me a chance to converse with others and decrease the feeling of loneliness.

In case you are not familiar with the benefits of yoga for a cancer patient, it encompasses stretching and deep breathing in each session. Yoga is often recommended for people with cancer because it can be a stress reliever and known for improving sleep and fatigue.

Togetherness matters.

It felt comforting for me to be around other people who were also going through similar circumstances and the things they were doing on their healing journey. For example, one survivor did catering and event planning for cancer survivors, where she would organize the location to host the activity, party favors, and healthy meals.

Another survivor knitted hats and socks to give out to survivors going through treatment or who had lost all of their hair. The items were warm and comfortable on the days when they were most needed.

While driving from work, I noticed the large black letters on a marquee that read, "Prayer Works." I wanted to explore this place more. I yearned to hear those words more now than ever before.

My children and I submerged ourselves in the church we'd found. The experience helped alleviate the hurt and distress. We took comfort in the knowledge that there was a higher power than ourselves. Church provided comfort to our souls.

Habits matter.

Once treatment was complete, I wanted to put the whole matter behind me and started to look closely at my overall health and wellness. Changing unhealthy habits like fast food in my diet, being more active and less sedentary were the first areas I would tackle. Studies have shown with proper nutrition, exercise, and controlling weight, survivors can help reduce the risk of cancer reoccurrence.

Some scientists believe a plant-based diet reduces the risk of cancer in general. Some even contend a diet of fresh fruits and vegetables with little meat and animal fat can lower the rates in some cancers like lung, breast, colon, and stomach.

Research finds eating red meat creates inflammation in the tissue and stimulates tumor growth in cancers. Plant foods contain antioxidants, vitamins A, C, and E and act as protection from free radicals - molecules that do damage to healthy cells. Fruits, nuts, and vegetables that contain phytochemicals stop the development of cancer.

A great deal of evidence points toward being overweight as a risk factor for different types of cancers. Chemotherapy can make some cancer patients lose weight because of a loss of appetite, anxiety, and the stress behind it. A dietician can aid in this matter and create a healthy diet and meal plan for you. It could mean just simply asking your doctor for some referrals.

In my research, these are some guidelines established for maintaining a healthy diet for breast cancer survivors:

- Eat five servings of fruits and vegetables each day. Servings are usually a cup-sized amount of greens or berries and a medium-sized piece of fruit. Only use plant-based seasoning like parsley or turmeric to add flavor to foods.

- Include whole-grain bread and cereals which would include brown rice, barley, bulgur, and oats. Avoid cakes, donuts, and white bread that are typically high in sugar.

- Choose lean proteins and avoid red or processed meats. Select fish, poultry, and tofu instead.

- Pick low-fat dairy products like low-fat milk instead of whole milk, which contains less fat. Consume skim milk, low-fat yogurt, and low-fat cheeses.

- A meal incorporating salmon, sardines, or canned tuna at least twice a week and a serving of whole grains like walnuts or flaxseeds.

- Avoid or limit alcohol usage. Some studies show a link between alcohol and cancer. Men should have no more than two drinks a day, and women one drink a day.

- Consuming Vitamin D has shown promise in the reduction of cancers to improve survival rates. These foods include salmon, sardines, fortified orange juice, milk, and cereals.

- Research studies are mixed on whether organic or nonorganic diets are most beneficial in preventing cancer or preventing the recurrence of cancer. Mostly, it is used to provide relief from some side effects and symptoms of cancer.

The use of alternative treatments and medicines can provide some relief from certain cancer side-effects and symptoms.

There are around 10 options in the category that are generally safe.

Sometimes cancer may make a survivor feel not in control of their health while alternative treatments can offer a certain level of control.

For example, these are alternative therapies to aid in your survivorship:

- To conquer anxiety, try hypnosis, massage, meditation, and other relaxation methods.

- To alleviate fatigue, participate in moderate exercises, massages, and yoga.

- To lessen nausea and vomiting enlist acupuncture, hypnosis, music, and aromatherapy.

- To ease pain, acupuncture, music, massage therapy, and hypnosis have shown to be beneficial.

- For sleep challenges, exercise, and yoga techniques help to relax the mind, body, and spirit.

- To help with stress, try a massage, yoga, hypnosis, exercise, and aromatherapy

I did try acupuncture, and it also seemed to help me with fatigue and various joint pain.

Acupuncture treatments involve the insertion of tiny needles into the skin at various pressure points.

Acupuncture can be helpful in alleviating nausea brought on by chemotherapy and stress.

Other forms of nontraditional therapies:

- Aromatherapy's focus is to create fragrances to aid in providing a relaxing sensation released into the air and oil applied to the body. Aromatherapy is most helpful in alleviating nausea, pain, and stress during a calming massage.

- Exercise helps to alleviate pain and fatigue brought on by stress during your cancer experience. It can prolong life in cancer survivors and increase their quality of life.

- Hypnosis has proven to be an effective technique performed by a certified therapist that aids in pain control, alleviating stress, and nausea symptoms from chemotherapy.

- Meditation and music therapy are also relaxation techniques.

- Supplements can help cancer survivors by strengthening the immune system, warding off diseases.

- Vitamin D is a good choice for cancer treatment and prevention.

- Antioxidants like vitamin A, vitamin C. vitamin E, and beta-carotene are believed to prevent cancer. Eating foods that contain these vitamins reduces the risk of cancer.

- Iron supplements to help to improve the fatigue brought on by chemotherapy and radiation.

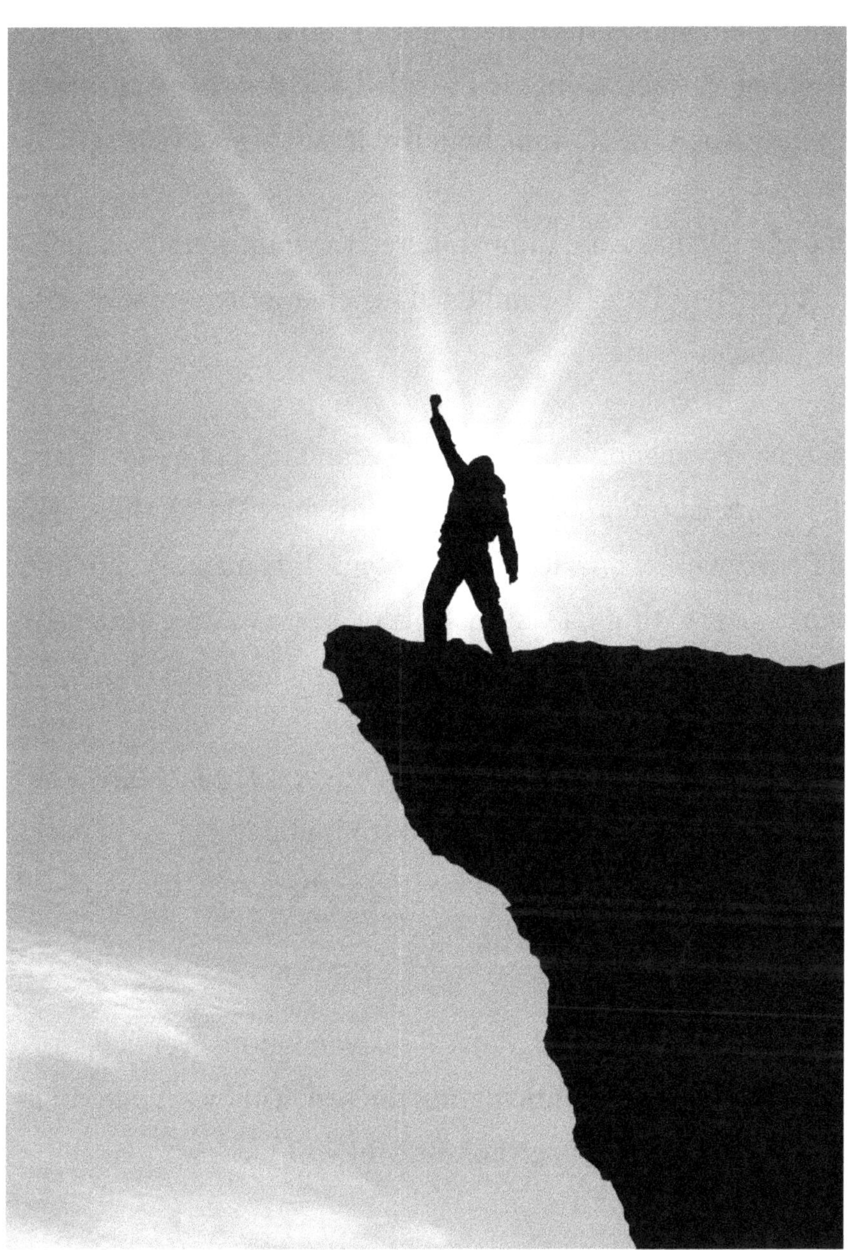

Twelve months into my survivorship, the time had come for surveillance and to take my annual mammogram.

As I waited and watched everyone in the waiting room listening for their names to be called, my nose began to sweat. Anxiety was at an all-time high like it had been a year ago.

For whatever reason, I remembered the faint sound of a bell ringing when I finally completed my chemotherapy sessions at the infusion center.

Hands were clapping all around me, and balloons were flying. It was a celebration of a successful mission. Maybe the smell of being in close quarters brought back this memory. I didn't know what to think. I was just sitting there waiting patiently for my turn to have the diagnostic test on my breast.

I wouldn't allow myself to think positively. The last time I did that, the rug was pulled clean out from under me, and I fell into a deep abyss, struggling to find something sturdy to hold onto, to pull myself back upright.

There should be a psychological session before every test to strengthen patients anticipating the test. That way, one could prepare themselves ahead of time for what was yet to come.

I counted the number of patients who were also waiting in the room to occupy my mind. I wondered what tragedy they were experiencing.

What were their lives like, and what had brought them here? Who knows we could be experiencing similar trauma?

You would think someone would reach their hands out to you in comfort and condolence. Each stood idly by watching patients disappear behind the closed front door.

Silence. Not one word spoken.

This was torture. I wouldn't wish this on my worst enemy.

Yet, I was thankful that the doctors had signed me up for a special program that covered all my medical expenses through this ordeal. I couldn't imagine having to deal with cancer and struggling to find ways to pay for medical care that would keep me alive.

People shifted in their seats as each person left the area to get closer to the door. I felt sick to my stomach.

My nerves were getting the best of me. Breathe.

Conversations I would have with various people like my boss, coworkers, friends, and family were, in essence, conversations I should have had with myself.

While I felt things were at a standstill, things actually continued to evolve around me. It felt somewhat selfish to only think of myself. I had never done that, so it was unchartered territory for me. Considering everyone else first had been the foundation of my life.

I thought about how I had allowed cancer to control me to the core. On a normal day, I would have been seeking a higher position at work, planning to attend concerts or upcoming shows, and looking for an adequate suitor.

Romance. Yeah, love or companionship would be in the mix. But now it seemed like a distant memory. I would be living my best life by myself. Who could I share these innermost thoughts with? I had to stay strong for my family despite being at my lowest.

The door finally opened, and the nurse holding her clipboard called my name and beckoned me forward.

Is this what it feels like at the end of the world? Are all your deeds written down and accounted for from the beginning of your life?

Thank GOD I learned how to repent for my sins early in life. As I walked slowly to the door, it dawned on me, I had been using cancer as an excuse for not going after those things I would have pursued.

I mentally blamed cancer for everything - my loneliness, my isolation, and my financial status. Cancer became my crutch. It gave me an excuse for not even trying anymore.

Still, no one is prepared to hear the big C word after a physical. The impact of the psychological and emotional toll that results from treatment and therapies that are required takes a major toll on the psyche and your emotional well-being.

People close to a survivor like friends and family may help from time to time in providing a warm shoulder to lean on. Even with that support, loneliness can still creep in.

Part of the loneliness stems from the fact that the breast cancer survivor is usually dealing with situations and emotions other people around them are not and cannot fully understand within the implications of the cancer experience.

My survival matters. Most of this is acknowledging the mental war that was waging inside my mind.

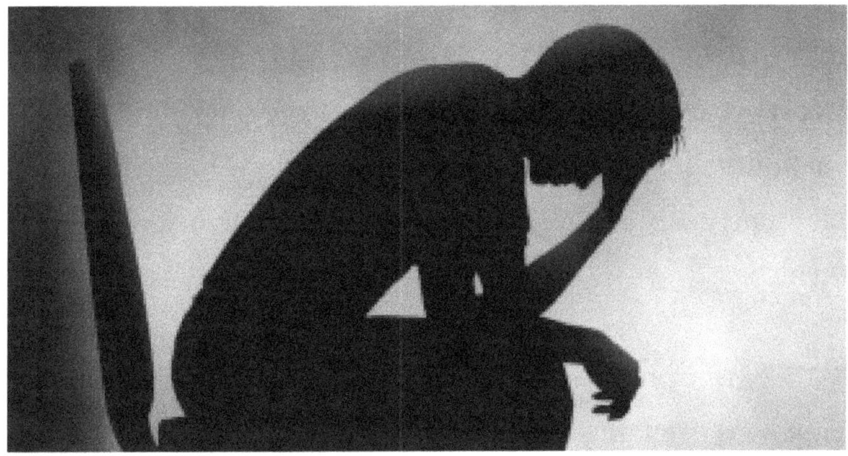

The struggle to communicate to others just how you really feel about the situation is difficult because it is hard for others to understand something they have never experienced.

Loneliness, especially chronic loneliness, may exacerbate the cancer experience. It seems like there is an overall sentiment after time goes by that the breast cancer survivor and others who are aware of the disease should move past the situation.

Some people may tend to distance themselves from you because of their own feelings of helplessness. Coping with the feelings of loneliness, helplessness, and depression may require professional assistance.

Some days I didn't even want to get out of bed. I would just lay there, thinking and feeling sorry for myself.

Image matters.

Breast cancer strikes at the very core of a female's womanhood. While the mastectomy saved my life, it took a toll on my body image. My body didn't seem to belong to me anymore.

Taking away physical attributes leaves little to hold on to. I felt empty. I'd used up everything I had to survive the diagnosis, the treatment, and efforts to move on.

I looked at the clothes hanging in my closet. There were some things I didn't feel comfortable doing anymore, like showing cleavage. Each blouse I picked out had to cover every top portion of my body. The type of clothing worn was important to hide the scars from the chemotherapy and the surgery. I always wore two shirts, covering any signs of scaring.

My paranoia of showing any parts of my body openly pushed me to purchase a slew of colorful scarves that I would wear around my neck. I wasn't attempting to make a fashion statement with the new look, but my thought was just to be able to move with ease throughout the day without confusion.

I was given a brochure that advertised a special clothing store for breast cancer survivors. Apparently, in this store the clerks measured and custom-made bras, underwear, shirts, and other clothing to compliment the patient. These items were made especially with the breast cancer survivor in mind.

As a customer of this store, I gained more confidence as I walked among others, at work, exercised, and otherwise went out in public. I didn't seem so consumed with concern over someone noticing. Before I found the store, it was like I was walking about with a scarlet letter glaring on my chest.

Being practical matters.

What I really didn't want is people walking around feeling sorry for me or feeling like they couldn't be themselves around me. So, with pen and paper in hand, I began my study on the impact of a cancer diagnosis on mental health.

Oftentimes, there is a major psychological impression of a cancer diagnosis. These are the facts:

- One in three people with a cancer diagnosis have mental and emotional distress.

- Nearly 25% of cancer survivors undergo symptoms of depression, and up to 45% experience some form of anxiety.

- Post-Traumatic Stress Disorder is experienced by many cancer survivors.

- Cancer survivors are over twice as likely to commit suicide compared to the general population.

- Adequately managing the psychological effects is central to surviving longer.

The physical and emotional scars the disease has left behind only show a constant reminder of the battle you just experienced. Even with going into remission, loneliness can linger. This can be intoxicating.

Sometimes the people close to a survivor can misunderstand the ramifications of breast cancer and how it has changed you. This is the prime reason why breast cancer survivors withhold the truth to others about what they are really thinking and feeling.

I had never questioned my mental health until now. Getting through the day as if it were business as usual became a chore.

My anxiety levels were soaring due to my breast cancer diagnosis.

Some studies have found people with breast cancer can suffer from Post-Traumatic Stress Disorder. This means they can experience symptoms of intense emotions as a veteran returning from war. This could affect a woman's quality of life in a negative way.

Seeking help matters.

When these symptoms began to persist, I decided to seek out a therapist. Talking openly about my feelings and utilizing her suggestions to connect to survivor support groups face-to-face really pulled me out of the psychological turmoil I was in.

We dialogued endlessly about the truth in my fear of cancer's recurrence. "Worry" is what the medical team called it. This was the source of my depression, feelings of isolation, and loneliness. I followed her guidance to the letter, and slowly things began to take a turn in the right direction.

I would recommend seeking the help of a therapist to assist with coping with the breast cancer journey. The mental health professional can show you steps to take to feel better and develop problem-solving skills. The therapist can help guide you along to think more positively about your circumstances.

See Appendix A for a list of mental health agencies that can help you find assistance.

My oncologist used to warn me about forgetting things that were once second nature. He called it "chemo-brain."

One day, all I could remember is that I forgot to wear my scarf that I wore faithfully draped around my neck every day. It literally was a security blanket as if it were used to ward off dangers or held magical superpowers.

I felt completely naked as if I were baring my riddled body to the world. In my mind, people could see the aftereffects from the surgery. They could see through me. Completely transparent.

I secretly would scan my body throughout the day as if something had changed or was altered right before my eyes. I was doing the same thing I had done to other people to myself, calling them paranoid about the way they felt they looked.

My internal thoughts were, "Get a grip, you are acting a little OCD-ish going over and over the same actions. You can't be beautiful unless you feel that you are such."

I would use my wit to distract people from looking too closely at my body. I didn't know I was the only person who saw the images of my ravaged torn body the way that I imagined them.

I could only imagine what the brave servicemen and women went through returning home from a treacherous battle hurt physically, emotionally, and psychologically with visible signs of almost losing their lives. They returned home to what must have felt like strangers.

No one could possibly imagine enduring such a feat. The people as you recalled them were the same. You were not the same, and those events that occurred in your time trumped the other daily experiences and struggles.

My high school sweetheart had enlisted in the military, and I longed for his safe return. When he finally returned to me, I pretended nothing was different about our relationship.

Oh, but it was. I looked closely in his eyes and could see there were things he could never reveal or recount the details of the harsh reality he had endured. His eyes seemed clouded. His innocence dissipated, and he was a stranger amongst us.

One thing I quickly realized was that most of the people in this world do not recognize mental illness as a viable cause for alarm. We tend to look at things from the surface and not what lay deep within our psyche - protruding thoughts and images that won't go away on its own.

He became angry and enraged over what seemed like the simplest things we both used to laugh about. I remember how he would drop everything when he saw me walk through the door.

Try as he might, he was not the man I fell in love with, and the relationship soon dissolved.

This could very well be me. Had I distanced everybody around who used to be a vital part of my world, or did they simply hold me at arm's length, not knowing what to expect from me?

Would I have to live with memories only and not personal life events in real-time?

Even in the midst of the struggle, I repeatedly thought there had to be a resource for people with past cancer experiences to meet other people who had undergone similar circumstances. I know staying alive was the top priory, but what a wonderful thing it would be to have someone to share in the struggle.

It was time to take action. I have always been the kind of person to create those things that didn't exist despite any backlash.

I did my homework and my research on creating such an entity where cancer survivors could meet and find companionship or friendship with the opposite sex for outings and travel exploits. This research took my mind off cancer for a while.

I didn't know it at the time, but it was part of my healing - doing something, being active, and being passionate about life again.

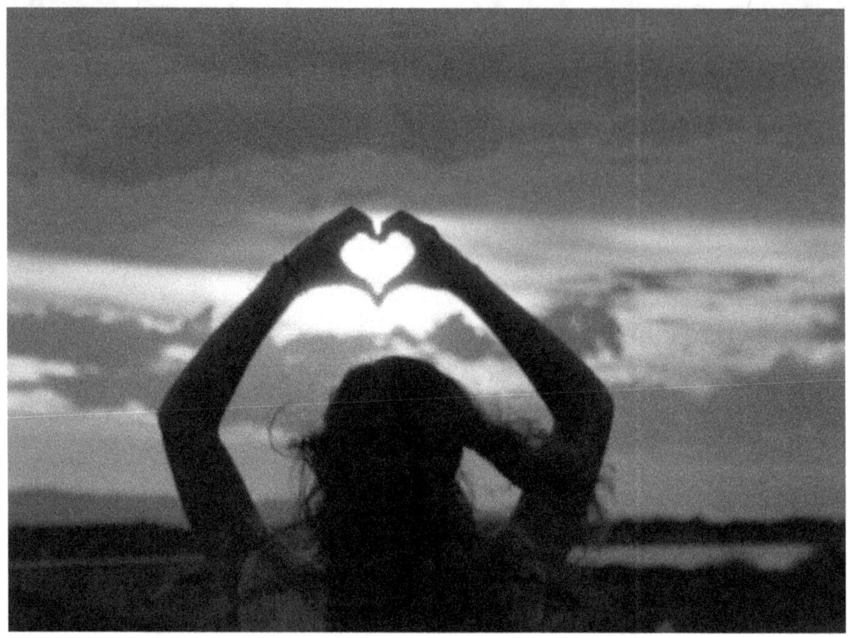

The worst part was over. The surgery, the chemotherapy, the radiation,and the hormone therapies were things of the past.

I just had to conquer the loneliness. Going through cancer battles alone was unacceptable. Surely, there had to be a resource out there to fill the gap.

I began intense research on the topic talking to other survivors without partners. I had specific goals in mind:

- To increase community awareness and support for people diagnosed with cancer.

- To make single cancer survivors feel they were not alone.

- To provide information and research to make the situation better.

- To open the door of opportunities to communicate with each other easily and quickly.

- To provide them a sense of togetherness to walk on the road as a team.

Let's face it, for most cancer survivors, the main priority is to get through treatment, be cancer-free, and lessen the ongoing worry regarding its reoccurrence.

After coming to grips with all of that, a realization surfaces that you are ready to enjoy some of the spice of life, to work out some of the kinks in your "new normal."

Cancer may have wreaked havoc on you emotionally and physically, but it didn't kill your spirit!

Deciding to date or to throw yourself into the dating pool can be a little unsettling at first. This feeling of apprehension is felt by most people, despite a cancer history, entering unchartered territory, meeting someone unknown.

Survivors tend to concentrate on what they consider their emotional and physical scars from their experience that they wear on their sleeves. In other words, it's like a shadow. It follows you wherever you go.

Nine times out of ten, potential suitors will come with a past carrying some level of physical or emotional scars from childhood or former romantic relationships.

Even before the diagnosis, treatment, or the road to recovery, a need to love and be loved is the very foundation of the human experience. Cancer doesn't change that.

Cancer survivors can feel more guarded in the areas of trust and sharing information about themselves. The cancer history may have altered trust, fear of rejection, and disclosure.

Facing with the realization of your own mortality is some pretty heavy stuff to carry around with you daily.

Other concerns could entail:

- Not meeting typical standards of beauty.

- Imperfect laws of attraction.

- They are somehow flawed or imperfect.

- They don't measure up against a traditional backdrop.

- Confidence is shaken.

- Overwhelmed by a plethora of "what if."

Everyone is different. Cancer survivors are a diverse group that is just as unique as the patients faced with various diagnoses and treatment options.

On the surface, dating may seem much like walking a tightrope. You never know when you might make a wrong turn or wrong decision and fall.

Keep this in mind:

First impressions are lasting impressions, so you want to put your best foot forward.

Find a place where you can get understanding and be yourself.

Some cancer survivors endure their experience without mates or significant others.

Survivors are a diverse group of cancer patients including the ones who are single. Even further, the single survivor is based on their own individuality.

Society tends to judge those who are unlike themselves for several reasons. Discrimination happens based on race, ethnicity, economic status, education status, gender, marriage status, skin color, sexual orientation, and yes, even health status.

Cancer survivors have one main thing in common, and that is to gain control over their lives and their bodies. Programs should be created to consider reality, not a one size fits all populations.

Every cancer survivor is different. They are people who have decided to date and are looking for a mate who is caring, understanding, and sincere like other single people.

While finding someone with these things in common is a daunting task, survivors shouldn't give up on the quest. I had to seek out those communities where meeting someone removed the fear of revealing I had a health challenge.

Cancer survivors do not have to expect any more problems in searching for a date than people without a cancer history and can wait for a few dates before disclosing.

Single cancer survivors without regard to race, color, religion, sex, national origin, disability status, economic, or education status are a unique group of survivors who experience diagnosis, treatment, and recovery without spouses or mates. Struggling to find a romantic partner is a chief goal for most people and could very well be an essential element to their well-being.

This is what I know from personal experience:

- 40% of young adults and 15% of those middle-aged are cancer survivors.

- Cancer survivors are less often married or have partners.

- They face finding a partner after they have finished with their treatment.

Here are some of the issues single cancer survivors face in trying to find a partner:

- Negative feelings about their bodies.

- Questioning their sexuality.

- Concern over fertility.

- Receiving a negative response from a potential partner regarding their appearance.

- Disclosing their cancer past.

Connection matters.

Internet dating websites that cater to cancer survivors or health-challenged people are the best way to find someone with whom you identify. The goal is to join people who can understand each other's circumstances.

No one has to face cancer alone, whether it's through diagnosis, treatment, and the road to recovery. Connect with individuals who have similar past experiences. This is critical for cancer survivors, especially for those who are single and going through the journey without mates, partners, or a support network.

The feeling of loneliness, isolation, and plagued by being self-conscious about their body image are oftentimes by-products of a cancer past.

My aim is to make the road a little less rocky as you navigate your way to living the best quality of life. Preserving those attributes that you and all humans possess to love and get love in return. These are basic human qualities. And so are desires.

Major aftereffects of a cancer diagnosis are loneliness and isolation. There are organizations that are here to help change all that. These groups help to support and guide you through your cancer survivorship by connecting you with others who share your same experience.

Don't cheat yourself out of finding friendships, romance, love, and happiness. Cancer singles organizations are designed to provide an opportunity and a place where people can meet, communicate, and ultimately form lifelong relationships in a safe and unintimidating environment.

Whether a cancer single is looking to meet other fellow cancer singles for companionship or romance, there is a place for you.

There is hope in obtaining a potential partner. Deciding to date after treatment is a surefire way to get on with your new life after cancer. People who have had cancer may want to meet others like them. This is the driving force that binds many together.

Everyone universally dreads the "C" word from a doctor's diagnosis. Some initial responses are numbness to complete shock.

Mostly, it is a feeling of where to go from this point in their lives. Those with children and spouses may get help and go through the journey together while others unmarried or with boyfriends or girlfriends may walk the journey alone.

This special group of cancer survivors needs to know they are not alone.

For the most part, single people look for the same qualities as a single cancer survivor does - someone loving, understanding, compatible.

I am on a mission to provide advocacy, education, awareness on this issue. To also give leadership to inspire and support to cancer survivors and those persons impacted by cancer.

Cancer survivors are as diverse as their treatment and the cancer they have been diagnosed with. The perspectives of cancer survivors should not be a one-size-fits-all approach. They are as diverse as their particular cancer, treatment, and individual perspectives.

Whether newly diagnosed, beginning, midway, or at the end of chemotherapy, radiation, or surgeries, there are resources to help on the journey to establish the "new normal."

Cancer survivors are looking for a camaraderie of like persons joined together to express concerns or get questions answered where sharing doesn't have to be uncomfortable with people who haven't experienced the disease. They need to know cancer doesn't stop them from finding companionship, even marriage. Cancer doesn't define their femininity or manhood.

Cancer survivors are not damaged goods because of their physical challenges and may feel a little guarded about opening up about sharing personal information about themselves and wonder how and when to reveal to potential mates about their cancer past.

According to the National Cancer Institute, about 42% of the adults aged 20 and older in the United States, nearly 700,000 annually, are unmarried by the time they are diagnosed with cancer.

There are over 100 million adults who are single, either divorced, widowed, or never married, with more than 30 million of them living on their own, according to https://www.cancercare.org/ (2016).

Whereas early detection of the disease is best in order to regulate it, these statistics are alarming since, by being single, the patients have an inadequate support system to help them through the treatment stages.

I was diagnosed with breast cancer in 2016. Now a cancer survivor and warrior, back then, I found out there were few avenues for single survivors to be able to connect and share their experiences and help each other cope with the diagnosis and treatments. While trying to search for my "new normal" as a single person, it came to me there may be others going through what I went through who are in need of comfort and support.

I am on a mission to form a movement that seeks to simply offer company to the numerous cancer patients and survivors out there who are single. Getting a cancer diagnosis can make a person feel overwhelmed, vulnerable, and alone.

By joining me, I get to be your family - reliable partners that stand with you through the whole stressful process. I want to be able to offer a chance for emotional grounding, a measure of ease, and understanding.

Some groups can assist in informed decision making regarding the complex nature of medical treatments for various cancer types, having been specially trained to do so.

The cancer survivors offer hope and encouragement to patients that there is life post-cancer, that they can beat it and get on with living productive lives. They may also be affiliated with cancer specialists who provide medical advice to our members on the best treatment plans to take.

By keeping up to date with the current cancer statistics, treatment plans, and trends, you are in a better position to adapt the methods used to keep up with the changes and strides made thus far.

The goal is to have a further decline of cancer mortality, to have more success stories regarding remissions, and to sensitize people on the need to lead a healthy lifestyle and beat the occurrence of new cancer cases altogether.

Finding your soulmate is challenging for anyone, especially one with a cancer history.

What's Your Matter?

Thank you so much for reading my story. I hope that it has inspired you and given you hope in some way.

My aim for writing this book was to share my experiences with you and to let you know that your cancer diagnosis is not an automatic death sentence. It won't be an easy road, but it is navigable.

If this book has helped you in any way, would you please consider leaving me a review on the website where ever you purchased this book? Reviews can help my book gain visibility and reach an even wider audience.

Sharing information matters. Open communication about this disease can only help all parties involved in the process. I hope to continue my efforts with a second book to come out soon.

I wish you the best.

Appendix A: Mental Health Resources

There are many reputable hotlines you can contact for answers to questions about mental health or mental illness, including:

The National Alliance on Mental Illness (NAMI): 1-800-950-6264, info@nami.org.	National Institute of Mental Health (NIMH): (866) 615-6464.	Mental Health America Hotline: Text MHA to 741741.	Crisis Text Line: Text CONNECT to 741741.
NAMI Alabama namialabama.org	NAMI Alaska namialaska.org	NAMI Arizona namiarizona.org	NAMI Arkansas namiarkansas.org
NAMI California www.namicalifornia.org	NAMI Colorado www.namicolorado.org	NAMI Connecticut www.namict.org	NAMI DC http://www.namidc.org
NAMI Delaware namidelaware.org	NAMI Florida namiflorida.org/	NAMI Georgia namiga.org/	NAMI Hawaii State http://namihawaii.org
NAMI Idaho http://idahonami.org	NAMI Illinois namiillinois.org	NAMI Indiana namiindiana.org	NAMI Iowa namiiowa.org

NAMI Kansas namikansas.org	NAMI Kentucky http://www.nami ky.org	NAMI Louisiana namilouisiana.or g	NAMI Maine http://namimain e.org
NAMI Maryland namimd.org	NAMI Massachusetts namimass.org	NAMI Michigan http://namimi.or g	NAMI Montana http://www.nami mt.org
NAMI Nebraska naminebraska.or g	NAMI Nevada naminevada.org	NAMI New Hampshire naminh.org	NAMI New Jersey http://www.nami nj.org
NAMI New Mexico naminm.org	NAMI New York State naminys.org	NAMI North Carolina http://naminc.or g	NAMI North Dakota http://www.nami nd.org
NAMI Ohio hnamiohio.org	NAMI Oklahoma namioklahoma.or g	NAMI Oregon namior.org	NAMI Pennsylvania namikeystonepa. org
NAMI Rhode Island namirhodeisland. org	NAMI South Dakota namisouthdakota .org	NAMI South Carolina namisc.org	NAMI Tennessee namitn.org
NAMI Texas httnamitexas.org	NAMI Utah namiut.org/	NAMI Of Vermont namivt.org	NAMI Virginia namivirginia.org
NAMI Washington	NAMI Virginia namivirginia.org	NAMI Minnesota namimn.org	NAMI Mississippi http://www.nami

http://www.nami wa.org			ms.org
NAMI Missouri http://namimisso uri.org	NAMI Wyoming namiwyoming.or g	NAMI Washington namiwa.org	MHA NW Arkansas mentalhealthame ricanwa.org/
NAMI Wisconsin Inc. namiwisconsin.or g	MHA Georgia mhageorgia.org	MHA Arizona www.mhaarizona .org	MHA Delaware mhainde.org/
MHA California http://www.mha c.org	Iowa mhadbq.org/	MHA Connecticut http://www.mhc onn.org	MHA Illinois http://www.mhai .org/
MHA Indiana https://www.mha i.net/	MHA Maryland http://www.mha md.org	MHA Hawaii mentalhealthhaw aii.org	MHA Illinois http://www.mhai .org/
MHA Montana http://montanam entalhealth.org/	MHA Nebraska http://www.mha-ne.org	MHA Kentucky www.mhaky.org	MHA Missouri https://www.mha -em.org/
MHA New York http://www.mha nys.org	MHA Rhode Island www.mhari.org	MHA Michigan www.mha-mi.com	MHA North Dakota www.mhand.org
MHA Pennsylvania www.mhapa.org	MHA Virginia http://www.mha v.org	MHA New Jersey http://www.mha nj.org	MHA So.Carolina www.mha-sc.org

Appendix B: Finding a Genetic Expert

Find out more about genetic cancers and the warning signs of hereditary cancer syndrome. You can learn about the different tests and what they can reveal about you and your family.

There are health care providers who specialize in genetics and will assist with understanding hereditary cancer risk. These specialists are called Geneticists, along with physicians, and genetic counselors are educated in the field of genetic training, holding master's degrees.

These are some ways to locate these specialists:

- The National Society of Genetic Counselors' website provides a searchable directory that lists over 3300 genetic counselors in the United States and Canada. Phone: 312-321-6834, Email: nsgc@nsgc.com

- Informed DNA is a network of board-certified genetic counselors who can consult with you by telephone. Face-to-face options are also available. Phone: 1-800-975-4819, Email: info@informeddna.com

- Grey Genetics provides genetic consultation by telephone. Phone: 1-516-900-4363, Email: info@greygenetics.com

- The National Cancer Institute offers a listing of health providers who specializes in genetic counseling and testing. Phone: 1-800-422-6237, Email: NCIInfo@nih.gov

- FORCE is an organization that provides a hotline at 1-866-288-RISK ext. 704. This helpline is comprised of volunteer board-certified genetic counselors who are available to answer questions on genetic testing and hereditary cancers. These volunteers will also aid in locating a counselor near you.

Bright Pink: Phone: 1-312-787-4412 Email: brightpink@brightpink.com
Focusing Our Risk of Cancer Empowered: Phone: 1-866-288-7475 Email: info@focusingourrisk.org
One In Forty.org: Phone: 1-508-330-8807 Email: allison@oneinforty.com
Pink Hope: Phone: 02 8084 2288 Email: info@pinkhope.org.au

Breast Cancer Resources.org: Phone: 1-610-642-6550

Living Beyond Breast Cancer: Phone: 1-855-807-6386 Email: mail@lbbc.org

Masthead: Phone: 1-855-233-5224 Email: info@mastheadpink.com

Sharsheret: Phone: 1-866-474-2774 Email: info@sharsheret.org

Sisters Network Inc.: Phone: 1-866-781-1808 Email: info@sistersnetworkinc.org

Susan G. Komen: Phone: 1-877-465-6636 Email: helpline@komen.org

Triple Negative Breast Cancer Foundation: Phone: 1-877-880-8622 Email: TNBChelpline@cancercare.org

Young Survival Coalition: Phone: 1-877-972-1101

American Society of Clinical Oncology: Phone: 1-571-483-1300 Email: customerservice@asco.org

Cancer Action Network: Phone: 1-202-661-5700

Cancer Legal Resource Center: Phone: 1-866-843-2572.org Email: CLRC@drlcenter.org

Coalition for Genetic Fairness.org: Phone: 1-202-966-8557 Email: sterry@geneticalliance

Department of Defense (DOD) Congressionally Direct Medical Research Programs: Phone: 1-301-619-7071 Email: usarmy.detrick.edcom-cdmrp-public-affairs@mail.mil
Friends of Cancer Research: Phone: 1-202-944-6700
Cancer Advocacy Now: Phone: 1-877-622-7937 Email: info@canceradvocacy.org
National Patient Advocate Foundation: Phone: 1-202-347-8009 Email: action@npaf.org
Patient Centered Outcomes Research Institute: Phone: 1-202-627-1884 Email: pfa@pcori.org
Research Advocacy Network: Phone: 1-877-276-2187 Email: info@researchadvocacy.org
No Stomach for Cancer http://www.nostomachforcancer.org/
Li-Fraumeni Syndrome (LFS) Li-Fraumeni Syndrome Association http://www.lfsassociation.org/
Lynch Syndrome/Hereditary Nonpolyposis Colorectal Cancer/Colon Cancer Alliance for Research and Education for Lynch Syndrome http://www.fightlynch.org/
Lynch Syndrome International http://www.lynchcancers.org/
Multiple Endocrine Neoplasia Association for Multiple Endocrine

Appendix C: Financial Assistance Agencies

The first stop for seeking financial assistance for breast cancer care is your local department of Social Services. This agency can help pay for utility bills, rent, mortgage, medical care, prescriptions, and food.

Beyond that, here are some agencies that may be able to offer help.

American Breast Cancer Foundation, Phone: 1-844-219-2223, Email: info@abcf.org
Assistance Fund, Inc./Cancer Copay Assistance Program, Phone: 1-855-730-5871, Email: HelpandHope@assistfund.org
Awesome Breast Forms, order@awesomebreastforms.org
Breast Friends, Co-Counseling Service, Phone: 1-415-828-2312, Email: conniesewing@breastfriends.org
Cancer Care, Copayment Assistance Program, Phone: 1-866-552-6729, Email: information@cancercarecopay.org
Cancer Care, Financial Assistance Program, Phone: 1-800-813-

4673, Email: info@cancercare.org
Cancer Care, Komen Treatment Assistance, Phone: 1-800-813-4673, Email: info@cancercare.org
Catherine H. Tuck Foundation, Phone: 1-888-411-5598, Email: infor@catherinefund.org
Christina S. Walsh, Breast Cancer Foundation, Phone: 1-723-853-7910, Email: christinabcf@comcast.net
The Compassion That Compels, Phone: 1-985-900-2009, Email: praying@compassionthatcompels.org
Donna Caneline, Phone: 1-866-236-6626
Feeling Beautiful Again Program, Phone: 1-936-231-8460, Email: info@iGoPink.org
Genevieve's Memorial Breast Cancer Recovery Grant, Phone: 1-516-500-3702, Email: mail@genevieveshelpinghands.org
Get a Mammy, Phone: 1-229-247-0753, Email: getamammy@bellsouth.net
Gouverneur Breast Cancer Fund, P.O. Box 64, Gouverneur, NY 13642
Hope Scarves, Phone: 1-502-333-9715, Email: hello@hopescarves.org

iGoPink-Breast Cancer Charities of America-Hope Fund Now, Phone: 1-936-231-8460, Email: helpnow@igopink.org
Impact One, Phone: 1-623-738-6794, Email: support@impactone.pink
KAMM Cares Foundation, Phone: 1-800-791-4099
Knitted Knockers, Email: fred@knittedknockers.info
Little Pink Houses of Hope, Phone: 1-336-213-4733, Email: retreat@littlepink.org
Lump to Laughter-Hope Packages, Phone: 1-910-617-4455, Email: info@lumptolaughter.org
Mama Marie Breast Cancer Foundation Survivors, Thrive Grant Program, Phone: 1-732-904-7885, Email: kristakaspere@mamacare.org
My Hope Bag, Phone: 1-480-987-0204, Email: info@myhopebag.org
My Hope Chest, Phone: 1-727-488-0320, Email: info@myhopechest.org
National Breast and Cervical Cancer Early, Detection Program, Phone: 1-800-232-4363
Patient Advocate Foundation - Metastatic Breast Cancer

Financial Aid Fund, Phone: 1-800-532-5274
Patient Services Inc. PSI, A.C.C.E.S.S., Phone: 1-888-700-7010, Email: uneedpsi@uneedpsi.org
Patient Services, Inc. MRI, Financial Assistance, Phone: 1-800-366-7741, Email: uneenpsi@uneedpsi.org
The Pink Daisy Project, Email: info@pinkdaisyproject.com
The Pink Pillow Project, Email: pinkpillowproject@gmail.com
Pink Heart Funds-Breast Prosthetic Program, Phone: 1-228-575-8299, Email: pinkheartfunds@gmail.com

About the Author

Celia Eloise lives in Central Georgia with her 4 kids Sadie, Susan, Sam, and Shawn. She is still cancer-free after 3 years. She hopes to give back by doing good such as volunteering in her community and lending an ear to other cancer survivors. She is also working on her second book.

www.ingramcontent.com/pod-product-compliance
Lightning Source LLC
Chambersburg PA
CBHW070714250726
48662CB00001B/410